The

Mediterranean Diet

Today

A Proven Diet

for a

Healthier Lifestyle

Ron Kness

It is no secret that obesity is on the rise, especially in the Western world! The state of obesity in the world today is a concern for all governments especially those in developed countries and with this comes the rise of heart disease and heart conditions.

And despite the efforts these governments have taken, the epidemic seems to become more serious. It affects both children as well as adults.

The main reason for the growth of this epidemic is lack of proper diet among the people. Most of the people have limited physical exercises as children spend a lot of time playing video and internet games or watching television.

Although this is a big epidemic, there is a solution… the modern Mediterranean diet.

Unlike normal diets, the modern Mediterranean diet is not a deprivation diet, meaning it is something you can stay on for the rest of your life.

The modern Mediterranean Diet is among the most established diets used for regaining health. It has been formulated based on scientific evidences conducted by experts in the field of medicine. Many individuals are currently using the diet as recommended by their physicians to achieve better levels of health.

In my newest book ***The Mediterranean Diet Today - A Proven Diet for a Healthier Lifestyle***, you will learn …

- **What the modern Mediterranean diet is (and isn't)**
- **The key to properly planning your Mediterranean diet**
- **The 14-day meal plan**
- **Practical advice on the best foods to eat on the Mediterranean diet**
- **How to live the Mediterranean lifestyle and keep fit**
- **A link to purchase all of the recipes in the 14-day meal plan**
- **Much, much more…**

This powerful guide will provide you with all the necessary information to easily transition you into living a healthy lifestyle and finally achieve your dream of dropping weight, keeping it off and stopping heart problems in their tracks … along with other health benefits of eating Mediterranean style.

Albert Einstein once said the definition of insanity is *"doing the same thing and expecting a different outcome."*

Now what I want you to do is think about how much you could change your life and your health ... your outcome - by doing something different if you really applied the strategies in this book. You could lose weight and keep it off while at the same time start improving your health. There are very few people who do not need to lose weight and get healthier ... especially as they age.

Or ... you can keep eating the same as you have in the past and continue to remain overweight while your health continues to decline.

The choice is yours. What are you going to do?

Published by:

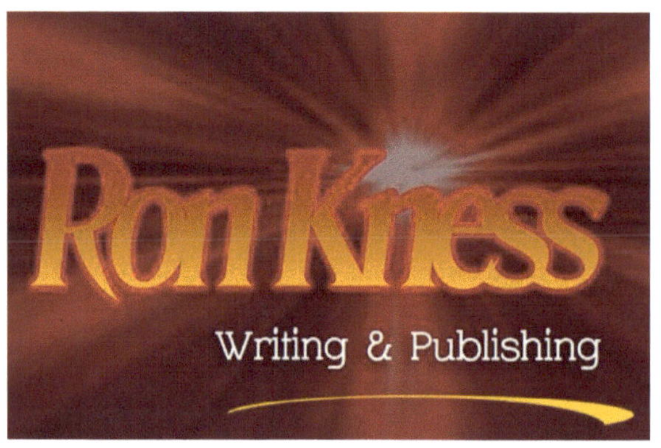

https://ronknesswriting.com

Ron Kness

Queen Creek, AZ

United States of America

for

Healthy Lifestyle Newsletters

ISBN: 9781703057270

Contents

Disclaimer

This publication is for informational purposes only and is not intended as medical advice. Medical advice should always be obtained from a qualified medical professional for any health conditions or symptoms associated with them.

Every possible effort has been made in preparing and researching this material. We make no warranties with respect to the accuracy, applicability of its contents or any omissions.

See your healthcare professional before starting any diet, health or exercise program!

Introduction

As the name suggests, the Mediterranean diet is a diet based on the traditional foods of the countries surrounding the Mediterranean Sea. Italy, Portugal, France, Spain and Greece are just some examples.

In America and the Western World, our diet has become increasingly high in fat and sugar. The red meat content is also extremely high – butter, sweets, cheese, burgers, steaks – you name it, we're eating it.

Unfortunately, this western diet is causing all kinds of health issues for the everyday man and woman. High cholesterol, diabetes, heart disease and even strokes can be caused by a high fat diet and our dependency on a convenient and fast food lifestyle is seeing a steady increase in these illnesses.

The areas surrounding the Mediterranean are home to the lowest rates of heart problems such as heart attacks, heart disease and other diet related health issues. This is largely because of their traditional diets. Don't get me wrong – some areas have started to adopt the Western diet of high fat foods and convenience eating but there are larger areas which stick to traditional foods and traditional home cooking.

When you think of home cooked meals you probably aren't thinking of the same kind of meals that the Mediterranean diet includes. In fact, you're probably thinking about bacon and egg breakfasts, burgers or takeaways for lunch and maybe slab of meat, potatoes and buttered veg for dinner!

For most people, this sounds like a great meal but it's not actually the healthiest way to eat. Research has shown that plant-based diets are actually far better for you than animal-based diets.

The Mediterranean diet though is a diet based on an entire region of countries as opposed to one cuisine. Generally, the diet consists of whole grains, dried beans and a huge range of vegetables and fruits as well as legumes. Small amounts of red meat are eaten but some people don't even bother with that.

If you're interested in learning more about the Mediterranean diet and how it can help you get on track to a much healthier lifestyle then this book is just for you. It's a personal guide through the Mediterranean diet and will help you get started as well as teach you some general health tips.

What Is the Mediterranean Diet?

Let's set the scene, shall we? The Mediterranean is a hugely popular holiday destination, probably because it's also one of the most beautiful places in the world. Rich history, culture and wonderful weather – it's no wonder people flock here in the hundreds and thousands every single year.

The cuisine is also one of the reasons people enjoy a visit to this part of the world. Not only one of the healthiest diets, Mediterranean cuisine is also one of the tastiest. A mixture of European, Asian and North African flavors can make for some very tasty meals.

Research has proven that this diet is one of the healthiest so it's sometimes a shock for people to learn that it can also taste really good. Even with so many countries playing a part in influencing the Mediterranean diet, they all have things in common which is why it's an interesting diet to consider.

It's not only the food. The attitude towards food is very different in the Med compared to the rest of the world. A lot of this is due to cultural differences and the ways in which they lead their lifestyles compared with America and the Western World.

A major part of the Mediterranean diet revolves around harvest and fresh food. Usually, the foods eaten are seasonal and are enjoyed shortly after they are harvested and not only that, but they don't travel far. Seasonal food is one aspect – the other is locality. The idea is that because food isn't transported far – it doesn't need any extra protection or preservatives. It's fresh from the field or orchard.

Vegetables in spring, tomatoes, cantaloupes, eggplants and watermelons in the summer! All fresh and seasonal vegetables and fruits. After summer, they work on wine pressing and olive harvests. You'll discover in this guide how all this plays a part in following the Mediterranean diet.

The lifestyle in the Med is perfect for outdoor markets – you might think you know what these are but until you've seen real fresh produce, you really don't.

In the USA, and other parts of the world where food is more processed and travels hundreds of miles before it's put up for sale, it suffers from what can only be described as dull looking food. In the Mediterranean, outdoor markets are exceptionally vibrant and colorful.

When it comes to meat, the Med diet is usually made up of lamb and veal or similar –
and usually only on special occasions. Meat isn't a huge part of the diet, but you will see
chicken and fish a lot in main courses.

Bread is something that not everyone would classify as healthy. However, you are
probably thinking of the white processed breads we have in the Western world. In Italy
for example, where the Med diet is traditional, they eat bread all the time. However, the
bread they eat is dark, whole grain bread with seeds and other additions – not like the
processed breads we see in our supermarkets.

You'll also find pasta and legumes are very popular with the Med diet. Legumes are
more affordable than meat so usually provide a great substitute. Lentils, chickpeas and
small red cranberry beans and even fava beans are super popular choices.

Cheese is a common option before and after meals but not in the same way we do over
here. Wine is also very commonly consumed with meals – but very few people drink for
recreation. Wine is almost always only enjoyed with meals.

Like we touched on earlier, the Mediterranean diet and way of life is simply different
because of their culture. You will find a way of life that is entirely different to ours. Food
is a social thing and involves massive families gathering and enjoying flavors and they
appreciate food far more than we do. It's an event and it's an enjoyable feast that
everyone can enjoy.

The History of the Mediterranean Diet

Back in the 1950s, research began to show that what we were eating in America wasn't as healthy as we'd all thought. Most of the dinners in America consisted of steak, potatoes and buttered rolls. Milk was also a very common drink with a meal.

This was because it was thought to be the nutritious way to eat. However, research started to show that the Mediterranean diet was actually a much healthier way of eating. Plant-based diets were far better for us and the lower rates of health problems in these parts of the world started to be understood.

The lower servings of red meat, higher quantities of fresh produce and fresh ingredients for home cooked meals mean a much healthier way of life. People from the Med tend to live much longer due to their better healthy-eating diet.

The biggest and most notable research into the Mediterranean diet came in the form of the Seven Countries Study by Ancel Keys in the 1950s and 1960s. This included a sample population from Greece, Italy, the former Yugoslavia, Finland, the Netherlands, Japan and the United States.

Specifically, the study explored the relationship between disease and diet. It involved over 12,000 men between the ages of 40 and 59. The study revealed that men on the Mediterranean diet were less likely to contract coronary heart disease.

Later studies proved that a diet low in saturated fat reduces cholesterol levels and the risk of heart disease. The Mediterranean diet mainly consists of monounsaturated fat which is the good kind of fat that your body needs. This good fat is mainly from olive oil which is a mainstay in most Mediterranean dishes.

Research continues to have a better understanding into the links between lower risk of heart disease and the Mediterranean diet. Apart from the diet, research now points towards increased activity as part of the lifestyle as another cause for this figure – so it's not all about diet but it's a huge part of it.

The Benefits of the Mediterranean Diet

So, we've established that the Mediterranean diet is definitely better for you than the usual American diet. However, let's take a real look at why and what the benefits of the Mediterranean diet are.

In basic terms, there are four major factors that play a role in your health:

- diet
- physical activity
- limiting alcohol intake
- not smoking

These four factors are major parts of what makes up a healthy lifestyle but the first is probably the most important. Our food is our fuel and it's exceptionally important that we pay attention to what we put into our bodies.

In terms of diet, traditional Mediterranean diet definitely has it all. Research has proven that the kinds of foods in this diet have a lot of benefits for your health. People under this diet have less chances of contracting metabolic illnesses like diabetes.

The same people also have less chances of getting inflamed cells which reduces the chance of developing diseases as well. Apart from less chances of coronary heart disease and other similar diseases, it has been shown that people on the Mediterranean diet also have a smaller risk of getting cancer. The same thing can be said about Parkinson's and Alzheimer's disease. Mentioned earlier and equally important is that people eating this diet live longer as well.

When it comes to fats, people tend to think that all fats are bad, but this is not the case. There are mainly two types of fats. Saturated fats come from animal products while poly- and mono-unsaturated fats are produced from plants, seeds and vegetable oil among others.

Monounsaturated fats are considered the healthiest and ideally should be included in your diet in place of other kinds of fat. The good news is that the Mediterranean diet revolves around this line of thinking. Of course, it is by no coincidence that this is the reason for the health benefits you get from it. All this is thanks to the kind of staple foods included in Mediterranean cuisine.

Mediterranean cuisine takes root from several countries each with its own distinct flavor. At the heart of these dishes though 20 are certain foods that have been proven by research to be important for good health. These foods for vitality are responsible for all the benefits of the Mediterranean diet and making you feel better at the same time.

Let's take a look at what there are in the next chapter …

The Mediterranean Diet Basics

The following foods are more or less a staple in any Mediterranean dish. You will find them in most recipes no matter what country from the region they come from.

Vegetables

No healthy diet is complete without vegetables. The truth is that you can never have too many vegetables in your diet. For better results, you want to make them part of your lunch, dinner and snacks as well. Apart from side dishes on your dinner plate, adding vegetables to your sandwiches can be very tasty as well. Essential vitamins and minerals can be found in vegetables which are important for good health.

Legumes

Legumes are an important part of any healthy diet. In botanical terms, legumes refer to a certain species of plant like beans. However, included also in this family are some nuts like peanut, soy and carob nuts, peas and lentils. These are great sources of fiber and protein.

Fruits and Nuts

Instead of munching on sugary sweets and other junk foods, a much healthier alternative would be to include fruits in your snacks. As such, it is important to stock up on apples, pears and oranges to always have something healthy to eat.

Drinking fresh juice is alright but eating an actual piece is a whole lot better. Nuts on the other hand have calories and contain good monounsaturated fats at the same time. Still, these are better taken in moderation because of their high calorie count.

Cereals and Grains

Whole grains are good for the health but making the transition from white and processed starches may be difficult for some. For better results, start with whole wheat breads from the lighter variety.

Work your way up to whole grain breads once you have developed a taste for whole wheat. Using this kind of bread for your sandwiches paves the way for a healthy and delicious snack. Other healthier alternatives include whole wheat pasta which goes with just about any kind of sauce you can think of.

It is the same story with brown rice as well. This increases your fiber intake easily. Consider replacing potatoes with sweet potatoes or yams as well.

Cereals which are less processed should be your top choice with oatmeal as the best example. Less sugar and more fiber is the goal here.

Fish

The Mediterranean diet calls for less servings of red meat and more fish in its place. With fish, you get a good source of protein without having to worry about getting bad fat like in beef and pork. In fact, you get the good kind of fat from fish with Omega-3 fats being the most important among them.

Studies have proven that Omega-3 fats help reduce the risk of heart disease. The progression of such a condition may also be prevented by eating fish or shellfish. Another thing is that fish is relatively more affordable and obviously a healthier source of protein than red meat.

Oils and Fats

When it comes to fats, olive oil is a mainstay in Mediterranean diet. It is a good source of monounsaturated fats which is the good kind of fat. This kind of fat does not increase blood cholesterol levels like saturated fats. Olive oil is also a good source of Vitamins A, B1, B2, C, D, E as well as K. Other healthy options include canola oil and grapeseed oil.

Olive oil is harvested from pressed ripe olives. The oil that comes from the first pressing is known as virgin. It is low in acid content with less than one percent concentration. This is regarded as the best of its kind with the fruitiest and best flavor.

Dairy

Traditional Mediterranean diet does not put a lot of emphasis on dairy products. In fact, people on this diet tend to reduce their consumption of dairy products. Even then, small servings usually of yogurt and cheese are made occasionally.

Meats

Like dairy, a Mediterranean diet calls for less meats. It is recommended to eat red meat just once a week with the average consumption of only four ounces on those days. When choosing meats, look for cuts that are leaner since these will have lesser amounts of saturated fats.

Alcohol

The same studies that explored the Mediterranean diet uncovered evidence that moderate consumption of alcohol is a good thing. Men who consumed two drinks per day or less had a lower risk of heart attack. But drinking more than this amount also showed a lower risk of heart attack as well. This finding even holds up when researchers took into account other factors, such as level of physical activity, age, medical history, body mass index and smoking.

In conclusion…

The health benefits from the Mediterranean diet all boil down to one thing: all the foods mentioned earlier are rich in essential vitamins and minerals that the body needs for vitality.

Consuming these foods can more or less guarantee that you are getting enough of these nutrients. Some of these are the following:

- **Antioxidants** – These help fight off free radicals which are chemical substances that roam around the body and cause damage to the cells.
- **Carotenoids** – This substance is found in red, orange and yellow plants, fruits and flowers. They help protect the body from damage caused by light and oxygen.
- **Monounsaturated Fats** – Also known as the good fat, this can help delay or reduce the risk of heart attack. Studies have also shown that cancer development is lowered as well.
- **Phytochemicals** – These substances can be found mostly in plants and are used for protection against bacteria, viruses and fungi.
- Overall, apart from reducing the risk of a wide range of chronic diseases, these above are proven to promote longer and healthy living as well.

The Mediterranean Way of Life

Apart from the food you eat, the Mediterranean diet calls for certain changes in your lifestyle. All this is to live a healthier and longer life. Compared to the American way of life, the Mediterranean one seems harsh and very stressful with little to none of the conveniences you are used to.

In a twist of fate, the Mediterranean way of life is much healthier than the American one. The modern life it seems is responsible for much of the health problems of today. Of course, it is very much possible to live a healthier lifestyle. All it takes is a little planning and adjustments where needed.

Physical activity has always been part of the Mediterranean way of life. People must exert a lot of effort just to grow, harvest and prepare food. This more than fulfills the exercise requirement for a healthier lifestyle.

It is not even seen as a requirement, just something that must and has always been done. This is in stark contrast to the American way of life and how exercise is seen as something expendable from the list of daily activities.

Numerous studies have shown that even the simplest forms of exercise can improve your overall health. In an issue of the ***New England Journal of Medicine*** published in 1999, it was revealed that women who got regular exercise reduced their risk of a heart attack by as much as 40 percent. Walking for at least five hours a week cuts this risk in half as well. Even exercises lasting only ten minutes, three times a day can have a significant impact.

Exercise has other benefits as well. Older people who undergo an aerobic exercise program will have better mental fitness than those who do not. Studies have proven that old people who exercised reacted 25 percent faster than people who did just stretch and toning exercises.

The benefits of exercise to the body are no coincidence. Science has proven that inactivity can result in more risk to chronic diseases, including heart disease, cancer diabetes and osteoporosis. The risk for obesity is reduced as well. Getting regular exercise also means better sleep, a more positive outlook and better overall health – mentally and physically.

Moving more not only prevents high blood pressure, but can lower it, if your levels are already high. And, it strengthens the heart making it work more efficiently.

At the same time, exercise prevents the spread of chemicals that promote atherosclerosis. With exercise, the body is better able to metabolize carbohydrates and increases sensitivity to insulin. This in turn lowers the incidence of diabetes.

With all these benefits, it comes as no surprise that exercise promotes a longer life. Studies have proven that even the smallest amount of exercise drops mortality rate significantly.

This is why an increasing number of physicians prescribe exercise for avoiding chronic diseases.

With the rigorous activity demanded by farming, most Mediterranean folk get their weight training exercise from this alone. It may not be the same as the weights at the gym, but it does have the same effect of strengthening your body.

This includes lifting, hauling, pulling, pushing, loading, chopping and digging among others. Evidently, strength training can become part of daily life without having to go to the gym. Strength training is somewhat different from other forms of exercises. For one thing, it needs less endurance and more short-term effort of increasing intensity. This builds both muscle and bone structures within the body.

Strong muscles do not just look better, they work better as well. Of course, this does not mean huge and hulking muscles. It means muscles that are fit, well-nourished and active.

Bigger muscles are better at processing oxygen which takes some load of the heart. Strong muscles around the joints also help relieve pressure around them. This added strength can certainly make a difference in daily life.

Don't have time to work out?

Is this really the case? With so much benefit from exercise, why not spare a few minutes of your time to get up and get going? Even the smallest of things can have a significant impact on your health.

Here are a few tips on fitting exercise into your busy schedule:

- Shorter but more frequent exercise sessions can be as effective as one entire session. The important thing here is to keep track of the total time and amount of effort exerted.
- Skip the elevator and climb up or down the stairs as often as possible. This is a great and simple way to get your heart pumping.
- To walk more, park your car as far as possible from your destination. This saves a lot of time and gas circling the parking lot for a convenient space.
- Do as much walking as possible. Surely going to the neighbor's house or the grocery does not need a car.
- When commuting, get off at least two stops earlier and continue the rest of the way on foot.
- In the office, get off your chair every fifteen minutes and stretch your muscles. A better idea would be to walk around the office for three minutes.
- If you keep missing exercising in the morning, try it in the afternoon instead. Some people are more energetic at that time of the day.
- Take your children or your dog to the park to play. How about a quick game of Frisbee while you are at it? This is definitely one of the simplest ways to exercise while having fun with your loved ones.
- In the same manner, try to convince a friend to exercise with you. This creates a support system prominently featured in the Mediterranean lifestyle.
- Instead of hiring someone else, consider doing your own household chores. Apart from getting exercise, you save money at the same time.

Planning Your Exercises

The American College of Sports Medicine recommended exercise of at least thirty minutes a day most days of the week. This applies for everyone regardless of age and fitness level.

For losing weight, aerobic activity of up to sixty minutes a day and strength training are needed. It may sound too much, but it is possible to fulfill this requirement with an exercise plan in place. This plan is quite simple and does not require any special skills, bulky gym equipment or special instruction.

Keep in mind that this is just a guide. The plan calls for exercise for three times a day, but you can perform a version for everyday use.

You have a free hand at adjusting the intensity level according to what suits you best. In terms of intensity though, be sure that you are working a sweat but not so hard to avoid straining your muscles.

Day One

- Perform gentle stretching of up to five minutes. To start your day, perform fifty jumping jacks or start with five first and work your way up to fifty.
- Get some fresh air and take a brisk walk for ten minutes during your coffee break.
- At lunch, take a brisk walk again for fifteen minutes. Climb up or down a flight of stairs before dinner.
- End the day with as many sit-ups and push-ups as you can add a few repetitions weekly. Finish off with some gentle stretching.

Day Two

This time walk in place briskly for five minutes but not before some gentle stretching. Commute to work but get off one stop earlier and walk the rest of the way. This should give you at least ten minutes.

- Walk around for fifteen minutes and eat a light lunch.
- For your coffee break, stair climbing would be nice.
- Finally, ride your bike around before dinner or do something else with equal intensity.

Day Three

- Start the day with gentle stretching and continue with five minutes of dancing.
- Take a brisk walk for twenty minutes with a few coworkers if possible.
- Instead of taking coffee, take two minutes to jog in place then perform ten jumping jacks and twenty wall push-ups. After this regimen, you will not need coffee anymore.
- More brisk walking for fifteen minutes wait once you get home after a light dinner. Why not take the whole family with you?
- If you have dumbbells or heavy cans of food, use this as weights against your chest while doing some sit-ups.

Coping with Stress

Modern living has a unique set of demands that can put a lot of stress in one person. Difficulties with finances, social relationships, careers and parenting are among the most common culprits. Over time, these demands develop into chronic stress and fatigue which is bad for the health.

Stress is a natural reaction of the body which is sometimes called the fight or flight response. It is actually a survival mechanism that has helped ancient peoples. It prepares the body to react quickly and get out of harm's way. Instead of dodging saber-toothed tigers though, modern man is presented with new challenges and dangers.

The stress hormones adrenaline and one that releases corticotrophin do certain changes in the body. Blood clumps together and plugs a potential wound and stop bleeding. The immune system prepares for trauma and muscles get a dose of blood sugar and stand ready. At the same time, heart rate and breathing increase.

Once the coast is clear, the body returns to normal thanks to cortisol. However, modern man faces so much stress that returning to normal is next to impossible. The result is a long-term condition that exposes the body to heart attacks.

Coping with Stress in the Mediterranean Way

In the Mediterranean way of life, people had plenty of ways to cope with stress. For one thing, social relationships with family and friends were kept strong and often prioritized. Even neighbors offered support for each other in times of need.

This kind of close support helps people cope with stress better. Another thing is that these people are closer to nature than most others. They grow and harvest their food off the land.

While there is not much conclusive evidence to suggest that nature reduces stress levels, anecdotal evidence suggests otherwise. There is just something in nature that puts the mind at ease.

Too much stress is bad for the health and this is unacceptable. The answer could not be more obvious. You will need to make a few changes in your lifestyle to weed out stress. Moving to the sun-drenched lands of the Mediterranean sounds like a good idea but is not really possible for most. You should know that it is possible to live a stress-free or at least a reduced stress life in this fast-paced world.

Consider the following tips as your guide:

- Appreciate your friends more. Try to improve your social relationships by keeping in touch more. Make it a point to ask family and friends their opinions and ideas. Joining support groups, organizations and other such groups is also a good idea.
- Meditation relives stress and it is a good idea to try it. The visualization involved can be enough to put your mind at ease and chase your worries away. Spend as much as ten minutes of your day to clearing your mind through meditation. How about imagining a relaxing stay at a traditional café in Southern France? Perhaps a stroll through the Greek coastline would do it? This is sure to recharge your mind and body and help you relax more.
- Step outside and enjoy the sun with the protection of sunscreen of course. Feel the breeze as it passes through gently and quietly. If you must, drive out of the city and towards somewhere with fresh air and enjoy your stay there.
- Consider things in context. Each stressful event, no matter what it may be, should be put into perspective. They may be inconvenient and irritating at times but your whole world does not need to come crashing down. Keep in mind that there are just some things you cannot change no matter how hard you try.

Starting Your New Mediterranean Lifestyle

Making the switch from your routine diet to a healthier one is a lot easier than you think. In this chapter, you will learn more about how to plan meals in the Mediterranean diet.

Keep in mind that this is just a framework to work with. It is by no means a strict meal plan. You are better off following a meal plan that suits your needs so be sure to make one for yourself. It is very much possible to lose weight under the Mediterranean diet.

For better results though, you want to consult your dietician for the best meal plan for this purpose. Remember that this diet calls for increased physical activity as well. You will need time to lie down, rest and relax too.

When making a meal plan, keep these guidelines in mind:

- Enjoy your food. - Remember that relishing every flavor of your food is part of the Mediterranean way of life. Beyond good nutrition, eating is a feast for the senses you must enjoy. It is not considered an inconvenient chore but an important part of life.
- Watch the servings. - In any diet, it is important for your calorie intake and activity level to breakeven. For weight loss, you want to consume fewer calories and move around more. Of course, this is easier said than done in today's lifestyle. Again, it is important to ask for advice from a dietician or other nutrition expert. In this meal plan, it is up to you to adjust serving sizes to meet your needs.
- Drink plenty of water. – As much as possible, try to drink at least six to eight glasses of water a day.
- Exercise, rest and relax – Apart from the diet itself, what you do in between meals is an important part of the Mediterranean diet. You should spend less time sitting down and more time moving and getting around. Go outdoors and find something to do to cover your exercise. Be sure to get enough rest and relaxation as well.

Conclusion

The healthier lifestyle in the Mediterranean proves one very important thing. Clearly, living and eating healthy is a choice anyone can make regardless of your current situation.

It is all a matter of taking the initiative to make the necessary changes to live healthy. With increased vitality, less risk from chronic diseases and a longer life, who would not want to?

This book has presented everything you need to know to become a healthier person through the Mediterranean diet. Now go out there and start applying everything you have learned here.

14-Day Meal Plan

If unsure about where to start as far as dishes for breakfast, lunch, snacks and dinner, I have included a 14-Day Meal Plan. Recipes for all the dishes noted can be found by searching the dish name on the Internet. However, if you would rather save the time of searching and get the recipes in a file, you can buy the Recipes PDF from me. It has a Table of Contents making it easy to find a specific recipe.

Sunday

Breakfast

A serving of Frittata made of 1 egg, 2 egg whites and ½ cup of sliced portabella mushrooms, 1 teaspoon of dill and ¼ cup of skim milk or water then mixed together and cooked with olive oil

1 to 2 slices of whole-grain toast

1 cup of low-fat and calcium-fortified soymilk

Lunch

A serving of Mediterranean Vegetables with Walnuts and Olive Vinaigrette

½ cup of White Beans with Cumin

1 small whole-grain roll

Snacks

A serving of Broiled Tomatoes

Dinner

A serving of Chicken Raisin Stew

A serving of Green Salad and Olive Oil Vinaigrette

½ piece of whole-grain pita pocket and 1 tablespoon of Tapenade

Monday

Breakfast

Eat 1 cup of oatmeal made of whole oats. Try this with fresh blueberry toppings and 1 tablespoon of raw walnuts.

Chow down this meal with 1 cup of low-fat soymilk. Drinking one that is calcium fortified is much better.

Lunch

Eat 1 pita pocket oh whole grain variety and filled with salad greens, 2 to 3 ounces of tuna and some mustard.

1 cup of red grapes

For dessert, try eating 1 cup of non-fat or low-fat yogurt of plain variety. Add 1 teaspoon honey or maple syrup.

Snacks

6 to 12 whole almonds and 1 to 2 whole wheat breadsticks

Dinner

Eat 1 cup of Tuscan Bean Soup with half a cup of brown rice.

2 cups of green salad and tomatoes with 1 tablespoon of Olive Oil Vinaigrette

1 serving of Cinnamon Oranges

Tuesday

Breakfast

2 pieces of small Orange-Banana Muffins

1 ½ cups of low-fat and calcium-fortified soymilk

½ to ¾ cup of berries

Lunch

1 serving of Sweet Corn and Toasted Walnut Risotto

1 serving of Macedonian Salad

Snacks

A serving of baby carrots with 1 to 2 tablespoons of Hummus Tahini

Dinner

A serving of Swordfish Steaks and Tomato Caper Sauce

A serving of Greek Salad

A serving of Wine-Stewed Figs with Yogurt Cream

Wednesday

Breakfast

1 egg and 2 egg whites scrambled with ¼ cup of skimmed milk, black pepper and fresh herbs

1 slice of whole-grain toast

½ grapefruit

Lunch

A serving of Gazpacho

A serving of Olive Oil Cheese Crisps

1 apple

1 cup of low-fat and calcium-fortified soymilk

Snacks

Caponata served with ¼ whole-grain pita pocket

Dinner

A serving of Ginger Lamb Stew

A serving of steamed broccoli tossed with minced garlic, hot pepper flakes and olive oil

½ cup of non-fat frozen vanilla yogurt with prune puree or berries for toppings

Breakfast

1 cup of whole-grain flaxseed cereal

1 cup of low-fat and calcium-fortified soymilk

2 to 4 whole pitted dates or prunes sliced into cereal

Lunch

A serving of Tabbouleh Salad

A serving of Sautéed Shrimp

½ cup of pineapple chunks

Snacks

A serving of Broiled Tomatoes

Dinner

A serving of Mediterranean Salad Sandwich with Harissa

Stuffed Peaches

Friday

Breakfast

¾ cup of Almond Couscous

½ cup of mandarin oranges

Lunch

A serving of Falafel with Tomato-Cucumber Relish

A serving of Green Salad with shredded carrots and olive oil vinaigrette

1 pear

1 cup of skimmed milk or low-fat and calcium fortified soymilk

Snacks

A serving of broccoli florets and dipped in 1 teaspoon of olive oil mixed with 1 tablespoon of

lemon juice

Dinner

A serving of Mediterranean Citrus Chicken

½ cup of spinach sautéed with 1 teaspoon of olive oil, minced garlic and 1 tablespoon of balsamic vinegar

Slices of apple dipped in 1 tablespoon of almond butter

Saturday

Breakfast

2 flaxseed or whole-grain waffles and sliced banana

1 cup of low-fat and calcium-fortified soymilk

Lunch

A serving of Moroccan-Spiced Cod

A serving of Beet Salad with Walnuts

2 fresh apricots and 1 cup of non-fat plain or sweetened yogurt

Snacks

1 sliced wheat bread with sprouts and 1 teaspoon olive oil

Dinner

A serving of Tuna Steaks with Green Sauce

1 cup of steamed green beans with minced fresh basil and ¼ cup of crumbled feta cheese

1 fresh nectarine

Breakfast

Grapefruit broiled with a sprinkle of brown sugar

1 scrambled egg with 1-ounce cheese topping

2 slices of whole-grain toast

Lunch

A serving of Ratatouille

A serving of white bean tossed in olive oil, fresh or dried basil and fresh lemon juice

Snacks

1 ounce of low-fat cheese and whole-grain crackers

Dinner

A serving of French Cassoulet

A serving of Green salad with Olive Oil Vinaigrette

Homemade custard made using skim milk or low-fat and calcium-fortified soymilk and berries for toppings

Monday

Breakfast

1 to 2 cups of whole-grain cereal with a handful of dried fruit and ½ ounces of dried nuts for toppings

1 cup of low-fat and calcium-fortified soymilk

Lunch

2 slices of whole-grain bread with 3 or more large leaves of Romaine lettuce, 1-ounce part skim mozzarella cheese, 3 ounces of low-fat turkey breast, a dash of olive oil and a little bit of salt and pepper

1 piece of fresh pear

Snacks

6 to 12 pieces of whole almonds and wholegrain crackers

Dinner

A serving of Moroccan Vegetable Stew

Couscous

A serving of Green Salad and shredded carrots drizzled with Olive Oil Vinaigrette

Fresh berries and ½ cup of soy ice cream in vanilla flavour.

Tuesday

Breakfast

Banana bread baked with olive or canola oil and whole-grain flour

½ ounce of nuts or seeds which can be mixed into the bread

1 piece of fresh orange

1 cup of low-fat, calcium-fortified soymilk with vanilla extract and a dash of cinnamon

Lunch

1 cup of pasta mixed with olive oil and topped with ½ ounces of walnut pieces, fresh parsley and 1 tablespoon of grated Parmesan cheese

A serving of Green Salad with Olive Oil Vinaigrette

Stuffed Peaches

Snacks

A serving of baby carrots and Hummus Tahini

Dinner

A serving of Tuscan Bean Soup

A serving of Macedonian Salad

1 to 2 slices of whole-grain bread

½ ounces of low-fat cheese

Wednesday

Breakfast

A serving of oatmeal or other hot cereal mixed with 1 to 2 cups of skim milk to cook and 1 to 2 spoonsful of pumpkin puree, a tablespoon each of snipped dried apricots, raisins, walnuts and a sprinkling of brown sugar

Lunch

A serving of mashed white beans and whole wheat pita bread

A serving of Greek Salad

A serving of Citrus Compote

Snacks

1 slice of whole-grain toast and 1 ½ tablespoons of peanut or almond butter

Dinner

A serving of Paella Valencia

A serving of steamed broccoli tossed in olive oil, hot pepper flakes and minced garlic

½ cup of non-fat frozen yogurt with prunes or berries for toppings

Thursday

Breakfast

1 piece of wholegrain bagel and 2 tablespoons of almond or peanut butter

6 pitted dates

1 cup of low-fat and calcium-fortified soymilk

Lunch

A serving of Mediterranean Vegetables and Walnuts and Olive Oil Vinaigrette

½ cup of pineapple slices mixed with ½ cup of plain non-fat yogurt

Snacks

A serving of steamed and chilled green beans dipped in Olive Oil Vinaigrette

Dinner

A serving of vegetable pizza with ½ ounces of part-skim mozzarella cheese

A serving of Stuffed Artichokes

A serving of Baked Apples and Pears

Friday

Breakfast

1 to 2 cups of whole-grain cereal, ½ ounces of nuts, dried fruit mixed with 1 cup of plain non-fat yogurt

Lunch

Whole-grain sesame crackers with Tapenade

Green salad with tomatoes, ¼ ounces of sliced almonds and Olive Oil Vinaigrette

1 tangerine

1 cup of low-fat and calcium-fortified soymilk

Snacks

Broccoli florets with a plain non-fat yogurt blended with low-fat cottage cheese as dip

Dinner

A serving of Seafood Risotto

½ cup of spinach sautéed in olive oil and mince garlic

A serving of grilled bananas

Saturday

Breakfast

Whole-grain pancakes made with olive oil and non-fat yogurt with ½ cup of fresh fruit, ¾ cup of non-fat yogurt and ½ ounces of nuts of your choice as toppings

1 cup of low-fat and calcium-fortified soymilk

Lunch

A serving of Falafel with Tomato-Cucumber Relish

Green salad served with Olive Oil Vinaigrette and fresh plum tomatoes

4 pieces of whole dried apricots

Snacks

1 slice of whole-grain toast with sunflower seeds and peanut butter as toppings

Dinner

Eggplant parmesan

1 cup of Italian green beans and oregano

Fruit salad made with fresh fruits

Books Referenced

Highlighted text in this book matches up to the words below. Following each word is a link to more information on that topic.

- Sugar - https://www.amazon.com/gp/product/1541232186

- Diabetes - https://healthylifestylenewsletter.com/diabetes/

- High Fat - https://www.amazon.com/gp/product/1536895792

- Heart disease - https://www.amazon.com/Heart-Health-Lifestyle-Putting-Factors/dp/1511940476

- Vegetables and fruits - https://www.amazon.com/gp/product/1535386053

- Lifestyle - https://www.amazon.com/gp/product/1546424660

- Plant-based diets - https://www.amazon.com/gp/product/1689839406

- Stress - https://www.amazon.com/gp/product/153978598X

About the Author

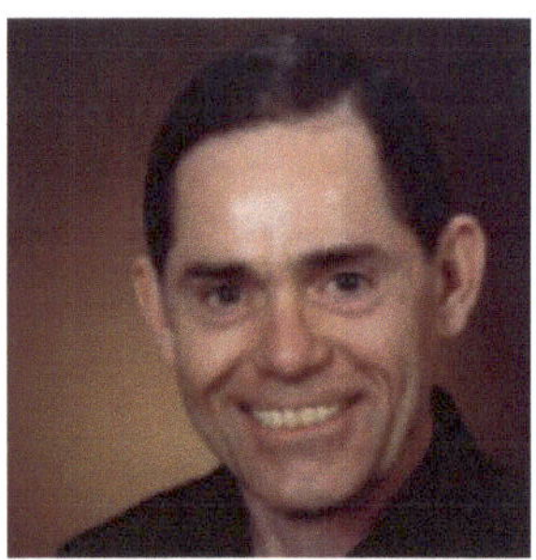

I have published numerous books on Amazon for Kindle and other publishing platforms. Both in electronic and POD formats.

While most of my books are on health and fitness in general, my topics of interest are leaning more toward aging baby boomers and the older population.

Besides my own writing, I also ghostwrite ebooks, books, reports, articles, blogs and do Kindle conversions for clients on a variety of topics. For a complete list of books, go to https://www.amazon.com/Ron-Kness/e/B0072M6PYO.

Today my wife and I are retired from our careers and live in San Tan Valley, AZ. I now write as a retirement business where you'll find me happily sitting in my office typing away on my laptop as I work on my next book or ghostwriting project . . . that is if we are not traveling on a cruise ship - our new-found mode of travel.